Second Edition

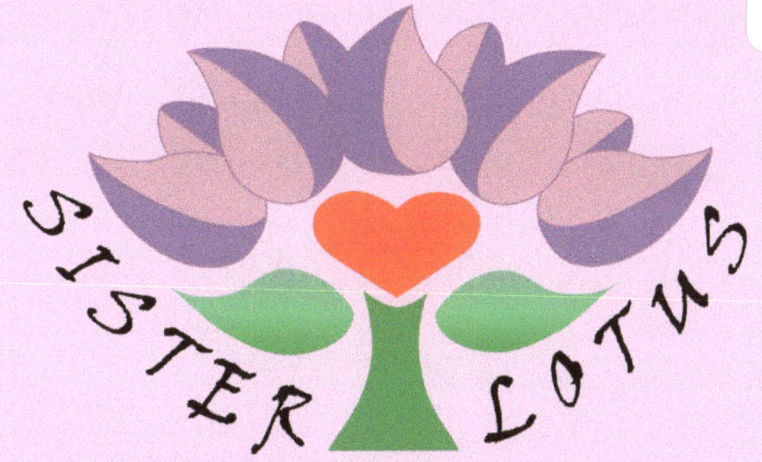

Yoga RYT-200 Apprenticeship Manual

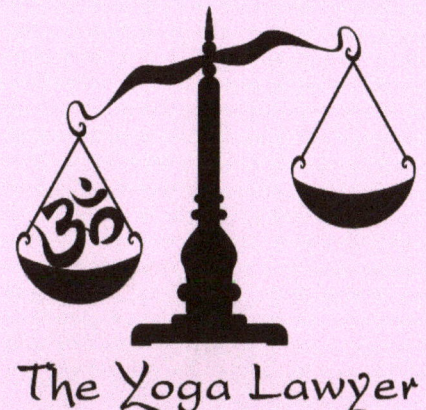

Copyright © 2021 by **Kelli Hastings**
2d ed. 2023

All rights reserved. No part of this publication may be reproduced, distributed or transmitted in any form or by any means, without prior written permission.

Sister Lotus Yoga, LLC
P.O. Box 531060
Orlando, FL 32853-060
www.sisterlotusyoga.com

RTY-200 Training Manual/ Kelli Hastings – 2d ed.
ISBN 978-1-7331173-3-3

The apprenticeship meets the Yoga Alliance Registered Yoga Teacher 200 (RYT-200) standards.

Contact Kelli Hastings:
kelli@theyogalawyer.com
www.theyogalawyer.com
(407)539-3032

Table of Contents

Table of Contents……………………………………………………………………………ii

Syllabus……………………………………………………………………………………...iv

Week 1……………………………………………………………………………………….1

Week 2………………………………………………………………………………………..2

Week 3………………………………………………………………………………………..6

Week 4………………………………………………………………………………………..7

Week 5……………………………………………………………………………………...10

Week 6……………………………………………………………………………………...18

Week 7……………………………………………………………………………………...22

Week 8……………………………………………………………………………………...31

Week 9……………………………………………………………………………………...32

Week 10…………………………………………………………………………………….33

Week 11…………………………………………………………………………………….36

Week 12…………………………………………………………………………………….38

Week 13…………………………………………………………………………………….39

Week 14…………………………………………………………………………………….40

Week 15…………………………………………………………………………………….41

Week 16…………………………………………………………………………………….42

Week 17…………………………………………………………………………………….43

Week 18…………………………………………………………………………………….47

Week 19…………………………………………………………………………………….52

Practicum/Week 20..54

Student Evaluations..56

Outside Yoga Class Worksheet..58

Required Assignments..59

Notes..60

Syllabus

Week	Topics/Sessions:	Reading	YA cred.*
1.	Asana I, including sukhasana and savasana	Surya Namaskara, Ashtanga Yoga Practice Manual	TTP/PE
2.	Asana II, including sequencing, methodology, Ashtanga tradition and lineage	Ashtanga Yoga Practice Manual, Yoga Mala, Yoga Anusthana	TTP/PE
3.	Ashtanga Tradition and lineage continued, Asana III	Ashtanga Yoga Practice Manual, Yoga Mala, Yoga Korunta article, Yogasanagalu	TTP/YH
4.	Types of Yoga, including what is yoga? Eight Limbs/Intro to Yoga Sutras	Eight limbs handout, types of yoga handout, Yoga Mala, Yoga Anusthana, Yoga Sutras	TTP/YH
5.	Pranayama	Ashtanga Yoga Practice Manual, Yoga Mala, Sequencing and Pranayama handouts,	TTP/YH
6.	Dharana/Dhyana/Pratyahara	Miracle of Mindfulness, Yoga Sutra III.35, Dalai Lama quote, Meditiation handout	TTP/PE
7.	Chanting/Sanskrit	Ashtanga Yoga Chants Handout, Yoga Sutras padas I and II, Amma Statement	TTP/PE
8.	Yoga Sutras	Yoga Sutras	TTP/YH/PE
9.	Yoga Sutras	Yoga Sutras	TTP/YH/PE
10.	Yoga Sutras	Yoga Sutras	TTP/YH/PE
11.	Anatomy/Physiology/Biomechanics	David Keil and Paul Grilley DVDs	AP
12.	Anatomy/Physiology/Biomechanics	David Keil and Paul Grilley DVDs	AP

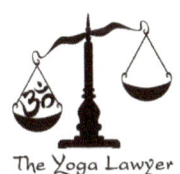

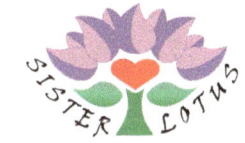

13.	Anatomy/Physiology/Biomechancs/Adjustments	David Keil and Paul Grilley DVDs	AP
14.	Bhagavad Gita	Bhagavad Gita	TTP/YH/PE
15.	Bhagavad Gita	Bhagavad Gita	TTP/YH/PE
16.	Bhagavad Gita	Bhagavad Gita	TTP/YH/PE
17.	Ayurveda	Handouts	E
18.	Business of yoga	Ethical statement from Yoga Alliance	PE
19.	Teaching Methodology	None	PE
20.	Practicum/wrap-up	None	PE

Books: Limited copies are available for borrowing. Some pdfs provided as indicated below:[1]

1. Sister Lotus Yoga RYT-200 Apprenticeship Training Manual by Kelli Hastings (included in cost of program, copy will be provided)

2. Ashtanga Yoga Practice Manual by David Swenson

3. Bhagavad Gita recommended version: commentary by Swami Satchidananda or Georg Feuerstein, but any version will work!

4. Introduction to Ayurveda ebook by Banyan Botanicals (pdf provided)

5. Miracle of Mindfulness by Thich Nhat Hanh (also available as an audiobook)

6. Surya Namaskara (pdf provided)

7. Yoga Anusthana by Sharath Jois (pdf of excerpts provided)

8. Yoga Mala by Pattabhi Jois

9. Yoga Sutras of Patanjali recommended version: translation by Mukunda Stiles

---

[1] The books on the list that are not provided are as follows: 2. Ashtanga Yoga Practice Manual; 3. Bhagavad Gita; 5. Miracle of Mindfulness; 8. Yoga Mala, 9. Yoga Sutras. For these books, it is recommended that you purchase or borrow a copy. Sister Lotus Yoga also has a limited number of copies of each of these that are available for borrowing and some may be found on the internet for free download.

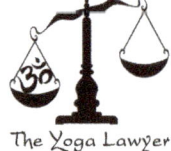

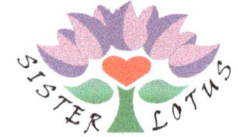

Videos (all videos will be provided):
1. Anatomy for Yoga with Paul Grilley
2. Yoganatomy 1&2 with David Keil
3. Hands-on Adjustments with David Keil
4. Breath of the Gods documentary
5. Yoga Short Forms with David Swenson

Each week there will be an assignment (including reading, self-study, and practice) and pre-recorded class or other videos. With the assignment, discussion, reading, practice, and self-study, the training will involve about 10 hours a week of time-commitment for 20 weeks, for a total of 200 hours.

We will arrange five (5) personal, periodic check-ins by phone, or video conference for personalized feedback.

There is also a private Facebook group and private online Website community where you can post questions and get feedback.

Cost[2]

The cost of the course is $799 in a one-time payment, or $177/month for five (5) months. The cost includes lifetime access to 20 weeks of online practices, class videos, assignments, and reading materials; access to private Facebook and Yogalawyer website groups for community feedback and support; physical copy of the SLY Training Manual; authorized individual access to copyrighted materials from some of the best yoga sources; five (5) personal check-ins with Kelli by phone or web conference; RYT-200 Yoga Alliance Certification upon course completion.

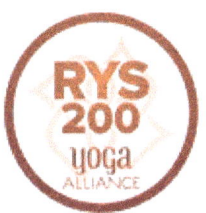

This course meets the Yoga Alliance Credentials as an "RYT-200" ("Registered Yoga Teacher 200-hour") teacher training. Upon successful completion of the course, students will receive a 200-hour RYT teaching certificate.

---

[2] If cost is any issue, please reach out. There are full and partial scholarship options, and no earnest yoga student should be denied yoga instruction due to cost.

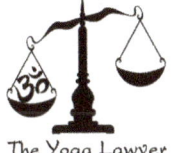

*Yoga Alliance Credentials Educational Categories

TTP – Techniques, Training, Practice – 75 hours – curriculum regarding Asana, Pranayama, and Meditation

AP – Anatomy and Physiology – 30 hours – curriculum regarding Anatomy, Physiology, and Biomechanics

YH – Yoga Humanities – 30 hours – curriculum regarding History, Philosophy, and Ethics

PE – Professional Essentials – 50 hours – curriculum regarding Teaching Methodology, Professional Development, and Practicum

E – Elective Hours – 15 hours – curriculum regarding Electives that are not part of the core RYT requirements

Total Hours: 200

The Sister Lotus Yoga RYT-200 Apprenticeship/Teacher Training Program will encompass all of the above categories of curriculum for a total of 200 hours. The week-by-week breakdown of which categories will be studied that week can be found in the above syllabus under the "YA Cred." Column.

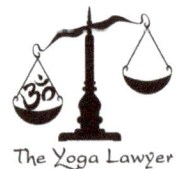

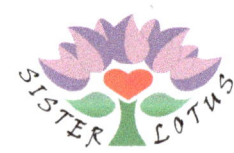

Asana I

Week One

Reading:

    Surya Namaskara by K. Pattabhi Jois (electronic copy provided), focusing on pp. 1-20.

    Ashtanga Yoga: The Practice Manual by David Swenson, pp. 15-19, 232-241

Practice: At least three (3) times this week, practice Surya Namaskara A and B three to five (3-5) times each, followed by the three (3) padmasana postures and savasana, or ask for an alternative warm-up if injury or physical limitation makes the sun salutations contraindicated.

Or, you can follow along with the Practice Videos, "Short (23-minute) Yoga Asana Practice" or the "Short Chair Yoga Session" at theyogalawyer.com/apprenticeship.

Assignment: (This will not be graded. Use this week's reading materials and internet to research)

1. What is "bhavana" and how can you apply this principle to your practice and this training course?

2. What does "Surya Namaskara" literally mean?

3. What is the metaphorical significance of the "Sun God"?

4. What are the meaning of the terms vinyasa, puraka, rechaka, drishti, and bandhas?

5. According to Pattabhi Jois, what medical conditions can be helped by practicing Surya Namaskara and other yogic practices?

6. What is sukhasana and savasana and how can they be used in your practice of Surya Namaskara and padmasana

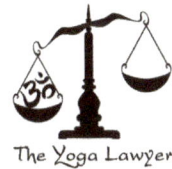
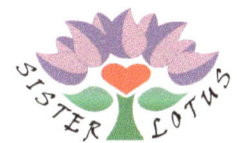

Asana II/Ashtanga Tradition

Week Two

Reading:

    Ashtanga Yoga: The Practice Manual by David Swenson, pp. 6-15.

    Sister Lotus Yoga ("SLY") Manual "Ashtanga Yoga," pp. 3-4

    SLY Manual "Letter from Sri K. Pattabhi Jois to Yoga Journal," p. 5

    Yoga Anusthana by Sharath Jois pp. 22-25, 29-34, 84-5 (excerpts to be provided)

Practice: Continue to practice at least three (3) times this week – practicing Surya Namaskara and your closing Padmasana postures. Also add in the respiratory postures from p. 85 of Yoga Anusthana to your padmasana postures.

You can follow along with the Practice Videos, "Short (23-minute) Yoga Asana Practice" or the "Short Chair Yoga Session" at theyogalawyer.com/apprenticeship

Assignment: (This will not be graded. Use this week's reading materials and internet to research)

1. What is Ashtanga yoga?

2. What does the word literally mean?

3. How would you describe the sequencing of Ashtanga Yoga asanas?

4. What is the "tristana" of Ashtanga Yoga? Per Sharath Jois?

5. What are the three bandhas?

6. What is Mysore?

7. What do Ashtangis typically do on new and full moon days?

8. How did Pattabhi Jois feel about "Power Yoga?"

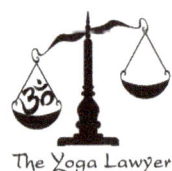

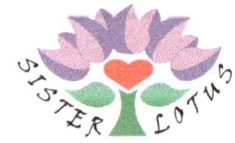

Ashtanga Yoga

At Sister Lotus Yoga, we teach traditional Ashtanga Yoga as taught by Shri K. Pattabhi Jois in Mysore, Karnataka, India. This method of Yoga has been handed down teacher-to-student for many thousands of years.

The teaching is very individualized, and takes into consideration the uniqueness of each student. While the focus is generally on yoga asana (exercises or postures), pranayama (yoga breathing), meditation, and other yoga techniques are also taught. The focus of the teaching depends on what the student is seeking from the practice – to get in shape? To gain strength and flexibility? To calm the mind? To connect with spirit?

Yoga asana is generally taught in the Mysore-style method, where each student is taught a set sequence of postures at his or her own pace. Each individual student's needs dictate how far in the sequence that student will go. As postures are mastered, new postures are added. However, class size determines how individualized the lesson will be. With larger groups, the lessons will be more broad and will tend to be more like the "led" yoga classes people are familiar with, while taking into consideration the uniqueness of the group.

Still, the tradition and lineage of the Ashtanga system are maintained. In Ashtanga yoga, students are not judged as compared to other students, because each individual student's practice may look different. It is a guided self-practice, where students are ultimately empowered to practice on their own, checking in with the teacher as needed for adjustments or additions to the teaching. This encourages students to look inward so that even the physical practice of asana becomes a moving meditation; a breathing exercise where the physical movements are laid upon the breath.

At the same time, beginners are not "thrown to the wolves," so to speak. When first learning, there is a lot of hands-on, individual attention until a student becomes firmly rooted in the practice. Do not be discourage by your perception of what people who do yoga look and act like. Anyone can do this yoga, regardless of body type, state of mind, age, level of fitness, level of flexibility, disability or injury.

The key to Ashtanga Yoga practice are three elements that help bring the attention inward, into the subtle energetic level of the body, while at the same time giving the practitioner a workout building strength, flexibility, and aerobic capacity. These three elements are breath, bandhas, and drishti.

Breath is the most important aspect of Ashtanga Yoga. The focus of attention should be on the breath. The breath is taken in deep and long through the nostrils while slightly contracting the throat to make a sound like the wind in the trees, or the inside of a conch shell. This is sometimes referred to as "ujjayi breathing."

The bandhas are "locks" that work both physically and energetically to move blood and prana (similar to the Chinese concept of "chi") throughout the body. The first and most important bandha is Moola bandha, or the pelvic floor lock. It is engaged by tightening the perineal muscles, between

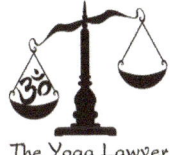

The Yoga Lawyer

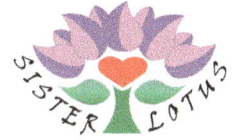

the genitals and the anus, like the sensation of stopping urination. Women may think of it like a kegel contraction. Moola bandha can be taken during the entirety of practice, with particular emphasis during the inhalation part of the breath.

Uddiyana bandha is found by contracting the lower abdomen. Think of pulling the belly button back toward the spine, partiularly on the exhalation part of the breath. Working together, with the emphasis on Moola bandha on the inhale and Uddiyana bandha on the exhale, prana is built up and pumped throughout the body. With the use of breath and bandhas, the Ashtanga practice builds internal heat and moves prana or energy in the body, thereby detoxifying the body from the inside out.

Drishtis are gaze points or focal points for the eyes. Every asana has a prescribed drishti, or place that the eyes should be focused. The main point of drishti is to focus the eyes and attention to a singular point, to help prevent the eyes and mind from wandering during practice. At first, it is more important to pick a comfortable gazing point and have the eyes focused there softly (not an intense stare), while working toward learning each of the prescribed drishtis for each asana.

The use of the breath, bandhas, and drishti help to direct the focus inward, into the more subtle levels of the body and make the practice more meditative than typical physical exercise.

Note that Ashtanga Yoga practitioners typically observe rest from asana practice on the new and full moon days. Our bodies are made up of mostly water and the moon, which also controls the tides, has a noticeable effect on our physical bodies.

Regular Ashtanga Yoga practitioners become in tune with their bodies and observe rest from asana on the new and full moon days, when the body typically is more susceptible to injury. A lighter practice, including pranayama and meditation can be taken on moon days under the guidance of a teacher.

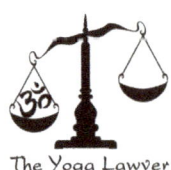

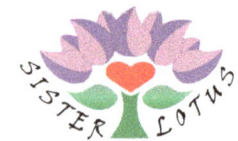

A letter from Sri.K. Pattabhi Jois to Yoga Journal, Nov. 1995

"I was disappointed to find that so many novice students have taken Ashtanga yoga and have turned it into a circus for their own fame and profit (Power Yoga, Jan/Feb 1995). The title 'Power Yoga' itself degrades the depth, purpose and method of the yoga system that I received from my guru, Sri. T. Krishnamacharya. Power is the property of God. It is not something to be collected for one's ego. Partial yoga methods out of line with their internal purpose can build up the 'six enemies' (desire, anger, greed, illusion, infatuation and envy) around the heart. The full ashtanga system practiced with devotion leads to freedom within one's heart. The Yoga Sutra II.28 confirms this 'Yogaanganusthanat asuddiksaye jnanadiptih avivekakhyateh', which means 'practicing all the aspects of yoga destroys the impurities so that the light of knowledge and discrimination shines'. It is unfortunate that students who have not yet matured in their own practice have changed the method and have cut out the essence of an ancient lineage to accommodate their own limitations.

The Ashtanga yoga system should never be confused with 'power yoga' or any whimsical creation which goes against the tradition of the many types of yoga shastras (scriptures). It would be a shame to lose the precious jewel of liberation in the mud of ignorant body building."

-K. Pattabhi Jois, Ashtanga Yoga Research Institute, Mysore, South India

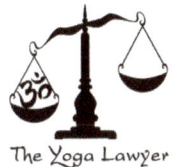

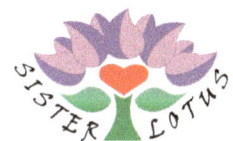

Ashtanga Tradition and Lineage/Asana cont'd

Week Three

Reading:

    <u>Yogasanagalu</u> by Krishnamacharya, pp. 1-11, 77 (copy provided)

    <u>Yoga Mala</u> by Sri K. Pattahbi Jois, forewards, preface, pp. 1-6 (stop at Yama), pp. 33-47

    "Breath of the Gods" documentary (link provided)

    <u>Yoga Korunta</u> article (copy provided)

Practice: Continue to practice at least three (3) times this week doing the sun salutations, the including the respiratory postures, followed by savasana.

You can follow along with the Practice Videos in the online course, "Short (23-minute) Yoga Asana Practice" or the "Short Chair Yoga Session" (also available at theyogalawyer.com/apprenticeship.

Assignment: (You will not be graded. Use this week's reading materials and internet to research)

1. Who was Pattahbi Jois' teacher? His teacher's teacher?

2. Who were each of the following yogis and, if deceased, how long did they live?
   a. BJS Iyengar;
   b. TKV Desikachar;
   c. Indra Devi; and,
   d. AG Mohan.

3. How are the above individuals connected?

4. What is parampara?

5. Look up the following important texts and familiarize yourself with what they are, who they are written by, and when they were written:
   a. Yoga Sutras;
   b. Hatha Yoga Pradipika;
   c. Upanishads;
   d. Yoga Korunta; and,
   e. Bhagavad Gita

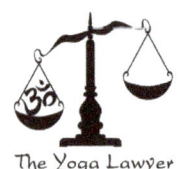

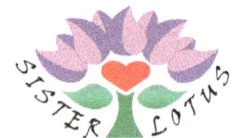

What is Yoga/Eight Limbs

Week Four

Reading:

    Yoga Mala by Sri K. Pattahbi Jois, pp. 6-31

    Yoga Anusthana by Sharath Jois p. 8-21

    SLY Manual "Eight Limbs," pp. 8-9

    "Six Yoga Systems" article (available in the online course materials)

    Yoga Sutras (check out Swamiji.com as an extra resource) read sutras I:1-4; II: 29-55; III:1-4

Practice: Continue to practice at least three (3) times this week doing the sun salutations, the including the respiratory postures, followed by savasana.

You can follow along with the Practice Videos in the online course, "Short (23-minute) Yoga Asana Practice" or the "Short Chair Yoga Session" (also available at theyogalawyer.com/apprenticeship).

Assignment: (This will not be graded. Use this week's reading materials and internet to research)

1. Note that the Yoga Sutras are divided into four (4) chapters or "padas." When you see "II:5" that means second pada, 5th sutra of the second pada.

   Upon reading the first pada, sutras 1-4 (I:1-4), how does Patanjali describe and define yoga?

2. You have read several descriptions of the Yamas and Niyamas as described by Patanjali, Pattabhi Jois, and Sharath Jois. What questions arise? How would you apply these principles to your life and yoga practice?

3. How many total sutras are there in the Yoga Sutras? How many sutras did Patanjali devote to asana? What do you think is the significance of that?

4. What are the names and meaning of the names of the four (4) padas of the Yoga Sutras?

5. Review the eight limbs and commit them to memory – not necessarily the Sanskrit names, English is fine. What questions do you have about the eight limbs of yoga?

6. Which limb does Pattabhi Jois stop at in the Yoga Mala? Which limbs does Sharath Jois describe at in Yoga Anusthana? Do either of them describe the higher limbs? Why or why not?

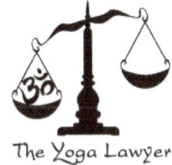

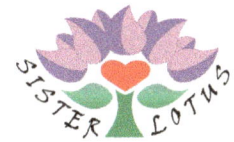

Patanjali's Eight Limbs

Patanjali's Yoga Sutras, written over 2000 years ago, offer an eight-limbed path of yoga called, "Ashtanga." Ashta means "eight" and "anga" means limb. Starting in Sutra II.29 Patanjali sets forth this eight-fold path as follows:

1. Yama (moral principles)

    a. Ahimsa – "non-harming." The sutras say that when we are fully grounded in non-harming, all hostility ceases in our presence. (II.35)

    b. Satya – "truthfulness." Being grounded in truthfulness, our actions and the fruits of those actions are also grounded in truthfulness and sincerity. (II.36)

    c. Asteya – "non-stealing." By being grounded in non-stealing, the sutras teach that all the precious things ("ratna" = gem) are gained.

    d. Brahmacarya –

        i. Brahma = the Creator, Supreme Being

        ii. Carya = "to live in"

        iii. "living in the Supreme Being"

        iv. Continence

        v. By abiding in brahmacarya, vitality is gained. (II.38)

    e. Aparigraha – "non-grasping." The sutras teach that upon the foundation of non-grasping, the reasons for birth are known. (II.39).

2. Niyama (observances)

    a. Sauca – "cleanliness"

    b. Santosha – "contentment"

    c. Tapah – "purification practice"

    d. Svadhyaya – "self-study"

    e. Ishvara Pranidhanani

        i. Ishvara = "the Divine" (our individual preference of the divine form)

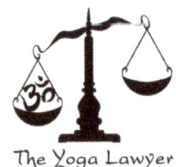

ii. Pranidhanani = "placed under the fullness"

iii. "placed under the fullness of the Divine"

iv. Surrender to the Divine

3. Asana

   a. As = "to be"

   b. San = "put together with"

   c. Na = "the eternal cosmic vibration"

   d. "to be put together with the eternal cosmic vibration"

   e. Yoga posture – 3 sutras:

      i. Sutra II.46 – asana is a steady comfortable posture;

      ii. Sutra II.47 – asana is the loosening of tension or effort and allowing attention to merge with the infinite;

      iii. Sutra II.48 – from asana practiced this way, duality ceases to be a disturbance.

4. Pranayama – "to bring forth life force (prana)", breathing practices

5. Pratyahara – sense withdrawal (senses may include the mind)

The first five are found in the Sadhana ("spiritual practice") Pada. The next three are found in the Vibhuti ("supernatural powers) Pada and are said to be internal practices as opposed to the first four which are external practices. Pratyahara is a mixed internal and external practice.

6. Dharana – "concentration." That is, the fixing of the mind to one point. (sutra III.1.).

7. Dhyana – "meditation." Meditation is the uninterrupted flow of concentration. (sutra III.2).

8. Samadhi – "bliss" or absorption in spirit. (sutra III.3)

9. Samyama – occurs with the last three (dharana, dhyana, and samadhi) flow together simultaneously

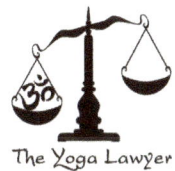
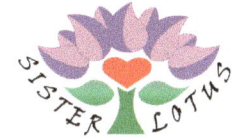

Sequencing, Pranayama, Eight Limbs

Week Five

Reading:

    Ashtanga Practice Manual by David Swenson pp. 21-27, 30-1, 34-41

    Yoga Mala by Sri K. Pattahbi Jois, pp. 48-57 (stop after Prarasita Padottanasana D)

    SLY Manual "Sequencing" p. 11

    SLY Manual "Pranayama" p. 12-16 (with illustrations of Ida/Pingala and Shanmukhi mudra)

Asana Practice: Continue to practice asana three (3) times this week. Let's add in some standing postures – Padangustasana, Padahastasana, Utthita Trikonasana, Utthita Parsvakonasana and Prarasita Padottanasana A-D. You can review variations of these in the Ashtanga Yoga Practice Manual by David Swenson. There is a new practice video – "Yoga Asana Practice with Standing Postures" on the course page.

Of course, you always have the option of staying with the Sun Salutations on your own or following along with the earlier Practice Videos, "Short (23-minute) Yoga Asana Practice" or the "Short Chair Yoga Session."

Pranayama Practice: Practice each of the pranayamas from the handout to familiarize yourself with them. They are pretty straightforward and you probably already have some familiarity with them. Do Nadi Shodhana, Sitali, or Bhramari (or any combination of these) five (5) times this week, even if only for five minutes at a time. You can do them before or after your asana practice and we can discuss the benefits of both methods. They are also featured in this week's class video.

Assignment: (This will not be graded. Use this week's reading materials and internet to research)

    Sequencing:

1. What are some other examples of possible "warm-ups" for our asana practice, other than those listed on the sequencing handout?

2. What are some other examples of standing, seated, and closing postures (fill in blanks on sequencing handout)?

3. What are some of the benefits of following a set sequencing framework?

4. What might be a disadvantage of following a set sequencing framework?

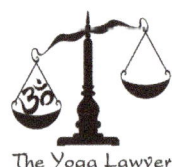

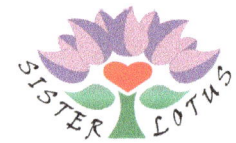

Pranayama:

5. Familiarize yourself with the terms "nadis," "ida," "pingala," and "sashumna" and look at the illustration on page 15.

6. What do you think is represented on the ida/pingala/sashumna illustration by the points where these 3 nadis intersect?

7. What might be some differences between regular breathing practices and pranayama?

8. Refresh yourself on the terms puraka, rechaka and kumbhaka and how they relate to pranayama.

Eight Limbs:

9. Notice ways to incorporate the eight limbs into your everyday life this week.

10. Pick one of the ten (10) yamas and niyamas, and write a short statement for personal use about your practice of it this week

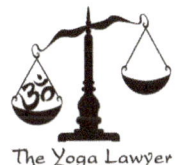

Sequencing

David Swenson's "Ashtanga vinyasa sandwich" p. 206, <u>Ashtanga Yoga: The Practice Manual</u>

First slice of bread:

    Warm up – ex. Surya Namaskara (Sun Salutations)
                Cat/cow
                Kundalini exercises (like spinning)
                Moon salutations
                _____
                _____

    Standing postures – ex. Padangusthasana (forward fold)
                             Trikonasana (triangle posture)
                             Parsvakonasana (side-angle posture)
                             _____
                             _____

Sandwich filling:

    Seated postures – ex. Paschimattanasana (seated forward fold)
                            Ardha Badha Padma Paschimattanasana (seated hip opener)
                            Baddha Konasana (butterfly posture)
                            _____
                            _____

    Twist – ex. Marichyasana (knee up, twisting looking back)

Second slice of bread:

    Closing postures –

        Backbending– ex. Urdva Dhanurasana (full back bend/bridge), Ustrasana (Camel), _____

        Inversions – ex. Sarvangasana (shoulder stand or legs on the wall)

        Padmasana – half, full, cross-legged or other comfortable position. Back to breath

    Savasana

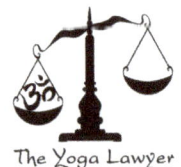

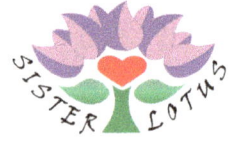

Pranayama

Pranayama is an ancient yoga practiced involving controlled breathing. "Prana" means life force energy, similar to the Chinese concept of "Chi." "Ayama" means to extend or draw out. Pranayama is one of the eight limbs of yoga taught in Patanjali's Ashtanga (eight-limbed) yoga system.

Use of pranayama techniques help us connect to the deeper reality behind our thoughts and may help quiet the mind. Pranayama also promotes balanced health as prana imbalances can be thought of as the root of all illness.

Nadi Shodhana ("nerve-cleansing") aka "alternate nostril breathing"

Notice how sometimes we breath predominantly through the right nostril and sometimes through the left. In a healthy individual, every minute or two, the breath shifts to the other side. The ancient rishis ("seers" who authored the Vedas) also noticed this, and discovered an energetic relationship between the left and right breath cycle. They correlated the breath cycle to the energy channels that run through the body, up and down the spine.

The left side is generally associated with male energy and the right with female energy. We can also think of it as yin and yang, sun and moon, ida and pingala (see attached illustration). All illness may be energetically traced back to some sort of imbalance between these two forces. Through nadi shodhana or alternate nostril breathing, we can bring these two forces into balance, thereby promoting healing of the body and calmness of mind.

The technique:
1. Sit comfortably on the floor or in a chair with feet flat (or lie down) with spine straight.
2. Breath in a deep normal breath.
3. Cover your right nostril with your right thumb and exhale through your left nostril only.
4. Keeping your right thumb on your right nostril, inhale through your left nostril only.
5. Retain your breath for a comfortable period and keep it the same throughout the practice.
6. Close your left nostril with your right pinky and ring finger and exhale through the right nostril only.
7. Keeping your right pinky and ring finger on your left nostril, inhale through your right nostril only.
8. Repeat steps 3-7 for five to ten minutes or as long as is prescribed by your qualified teacher.
9. End with an exhale on the right side.

Suryabhedha pranayama ("sun" or right nostril breathing)

Builds heat in the body by engaging right breath channel (sun channel/pingala). The technique is similar to nadi shodhana. Can be used in the winter or when cold.

The technique:

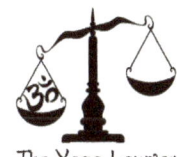

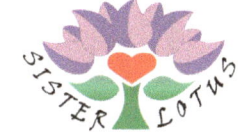

1. Sit comfortably on the floor or in a chair with feet flat (or lie down) with spine straight.
2. Breath in a deep normal breath.
3. Using the same hand positions as in nadi shodhana (above), this time inhale only through your right nostril and exhale only through your left nostril.
4. Repeat until sufficient heat is built or as prescribed by your teacher.

Candrbheda pranayama ("moon" or left nostril breathing)

Builds coolness in the body by engaging the left breath channel (moon channel/ida). The technique is the same as suryabheda pranayama except you inhale only on the left, exhale only on the right.

Take care with both of the above techniques so as not to create an imbalance in the body.

Sitali pranayama (cooling breath)

This is another cooling technique that is less likely to cause an imbalance than candrabheda pranayama. It can be used whenever coolness is needed or to balance pitta dosha.

The technique
1. Sit comfortably on the floor or in a chair with feet flat (or lie down) with spine straight.
2. Curl your tongue into a tube or lightly clench teeth together and press tongue up against the back of teeth.
3. Inhale slowly through curled tongue or lightly clenched teeth. You should feel cool air coming in.
4. Exhale normally or with slightly contracted epiglottis to produce a light sound.
5. Repeat until cool or as prescribed by your teacher.

Bhramari pranayama (humming bee breath)

This pranayama touts many health benefits, and may be good for transmuting anger and anxiety.

The technique
1. Sit comfortably on the floor or in a chair with feet flat (or lie down) with spine straight.
2. Breath in a deep normal breath.
3. Plugging you ears with your index finger or thumbs or do Shanmukhi Mudra (see attached illustration)
4. On your exhale make a humming sound like a bee as you slowly release your breath.
5. Repeat for several minutes or as recommended by your teacher.
6. Play with different frequencies of sound.

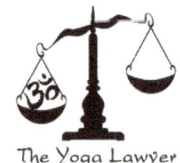
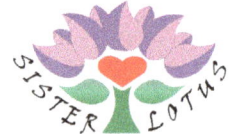

Three Main Nadis: Ida, Pingala, Sushumna

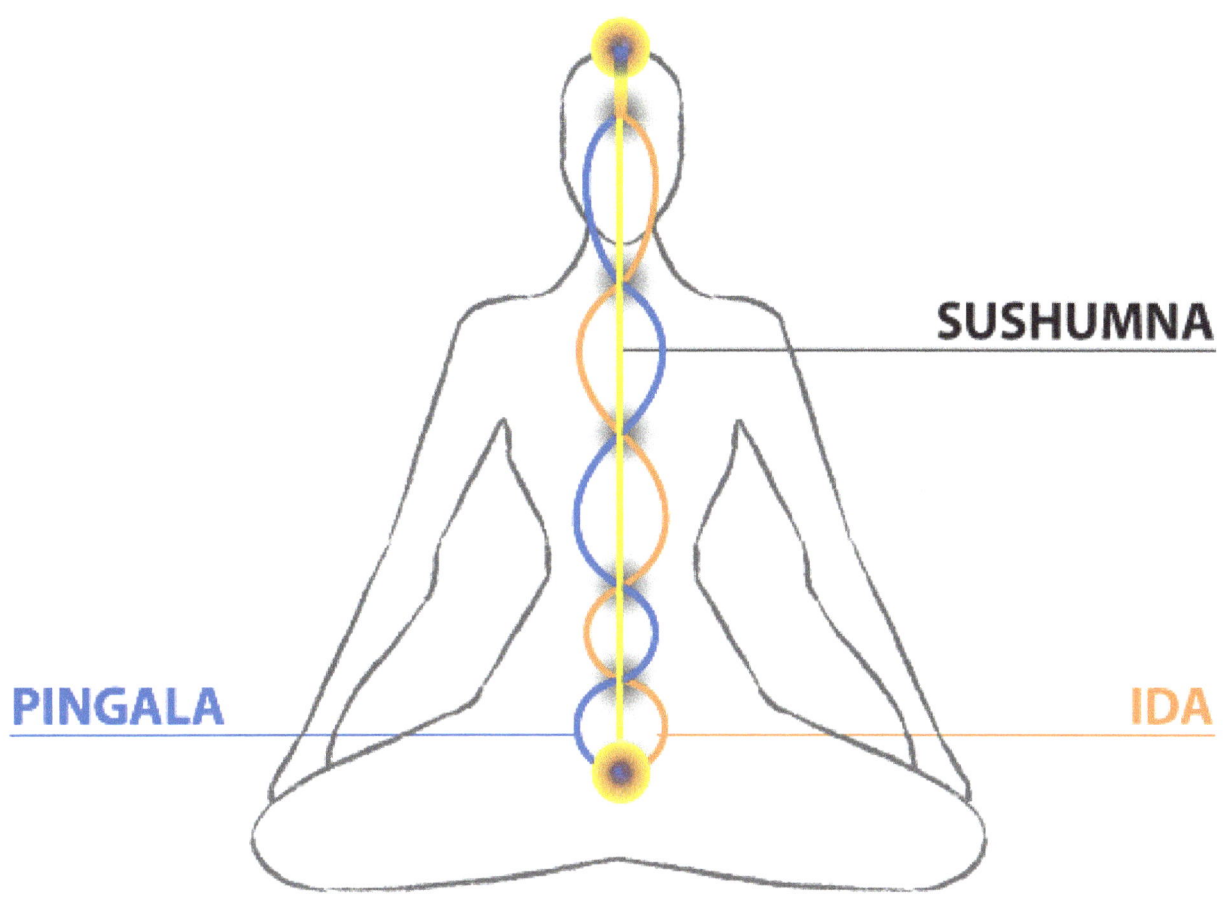

Shanmukhi Mudra

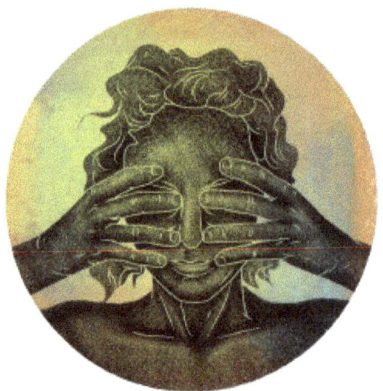

Shanmukhi mudra is a sacred hand gesture or "seal," used during yoga and meditation practice as a means of channeling the flow of vital life force energy known as prana. This gesture represents closing the six gates of perception – the eyes, ears, nose and mouth. The term is derived from three Sanskrit roots; shan, meaning "six;" mukhi, meaning "face" or "gate" and mudra, meaning "gesture," "mark" or "seal."

Shanmukhi mudra is typically performed in a stable, seated meditation posture such as Siddhasana (Accomplished Pose), Padmasana (Lotus Pose) or Sukhasana (Easy Pose). To practice Shanmukhi mudra, first raise both hands in front of the face with elbows pointing outwards, in line with the shoulders. With eyes closed, gently press the index fingers to the inner corners of the eyes, place the middle fingers on either side of the nose, the ring fingers above the lips and the little fingers below the mouth. Use the thumbs to gently close the ears. The spine should remain upright and the shoulders relaxed.

Shanmukhi mudra is usually practiced for five to ten minutes, often in preparation for meditation. This mudra is also known as Yoni mudra.

Shanmukhi mudra involves closing the ears, eyes, nose and mouth with the fingers, helping the practitioner to withdraw the senses and turn the awareness inwards. As such, it can be considered a practice of pratyahara (sense withdrawal), which is the preliminary stage of dharana (concentration) and dhyana (meditation) according to the Yoga Sutras of Patanjali.

For maximum benefit, this gesture should be accompanied with pranayama (breathing techniques) or bandhas (energetic locks). Shanmukhi mudra is commonly practiced with brahmari, a pranayama otherwise known as Bee Breath, in which the exhale is used to make a humming sound. In this technique, the mudra enables the practitioner to focus on the inner vibration created by the bhramari breath. In addition to heightening awareness and serving as preparation for meditation, shanmukhi mudra is credited with the following benefits:

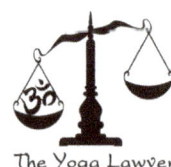
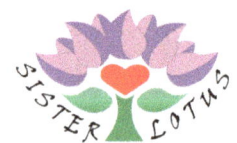

- Calms the mind and nervous system
- Relaxes and rejuvenates the eyes and facial muscles
- Balances internal and external awareness
- Creates a state of pratyahara
- Enhances focus and introspection
- Helps in managing anxiety

In the practice of Kundalini yoga, Shanmukhi mudra is also used as a means of awakening the kundalini (serpent) energy which lies dormant at the base of the spine. In order to achieve this, Shanmukhi mudra is accompanied with internal holding of breath, though this is an advanced practice and should only be undertaken with the guidance of an experienced teacher.

Above text from Yogapedia: https://www.yogapedia.com/definition/8752/shanmukhi-mudra

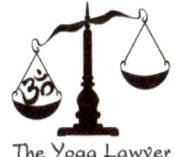

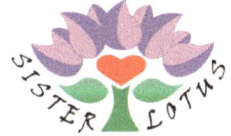

Dharana/Dhyana (Eight Limbs cont'd)

Week Six

Reading:

    Miracle of Mindfulness by Thich Nhat Hanh

    SLY Manual "Meditation," p. 20-1

    Yoga Sutra III.35 ("By practicing samyama on the heart, knowledge of the mind is attained")

    Dalai Lama quote "An open heart is an open mind."

Asana and Pranayama Practice: Continue to practice asana, pranayama, or a combination of asana and pranayama this week. For asana, keep working on the Ashtanga "sandwich," using the provided online videos or on your own. For pranayama, practice nadi shodhana, sitali, bhramari, or other pranayamas you know before or after your asana practice or on their own.

Dharana/Dhyana (Concentration/Meditation) Practice: Read or listen to the "Miracle of Mindfulness" and practice some of the mindfulness techniques described, like washing the dishes with mindfulness or walking the path with mindfulness.

Also read through the techniques from the Meditation section of this manual (below) and practice one or more of the techniques (or the techniques from Miracle of Mindfulness) several times this week, even if only for five minutes at a time. It can be done before or after your asana/pranayama practice, at night before bed, or any other time of day that works for you, even while you are doing other work.

Assignment (This will not be graded. Use this week's reading materials and internet to research):

1. Read or listen to the Miracle of Mindfulness and prepare a short paper (a few paragraphs to one page is fine) to turn in. In it, summarize the message of Thich Nhat Hanh's book in your own words, as if you were explaining the essence of it to someone who had never read it and had no meditation experience. This is one of a handful of "accountability assignments" that are not graded but are part of the course.

2. In your meditation/mindfulness practices this week, which techniques were you naturally drawn to or averse to? Was there a particular practice that came easier or with more difficulty to you? What did you observe about your experience of meditation this week?

3. Notice the difference between "constant" mindfulness and yogic practices (like washing the dishes mindfully) which can be practiced all day long and "sit-down" meditation/mindfulness practices which require time set aside specifically to practice a specific technique. What are some examples of each type?

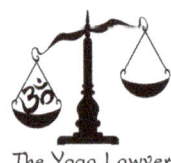

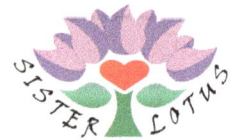

4. Contemplate Yoga sutra III.35, "By practicing samyama on the heart, knowledge of the mind is attained" and the Dalai Lama's quote, "an open mind is an open heart."

    a. How might mindfulness/meditative practices (i.e. Jnana yoga) relate to devotional practices (i.e. bhakti yoga)?

    b. How might devotional practices lead to mindfulness and vice versa?

5. Pratyahara – think about ways you might practice pratyahara (Shanmukhi mudra and floating are two (2) ways, though there are others).

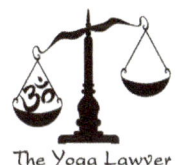

Meditation

Meditation does not necessarily mean a state of no thoughts. When you're meditating, you are being present or "mindful," and you're open to seeing the unity in everything. Sometimes this unity may come in the form of a thought. When you're not being present, you'll find your thoughts are more like an endless loop that play over and over again the same ideas – mostly recollecting the past or projecting into the future.

The point of meditating is not to stop your thoughts; it is to become aware of them; to become the nonjudgmental observer of your thoughts. Trying to stop a thought is hard. For example: try not to think about a pink elephant. Inevitably, you will think about a pink elephant.

The more you meditate, the calmer your mind will become. Human beings have amazing creative and healing capabilities when we are tapped into our natural, calm state of mind.

Simple Meditation Techniques:

Love meditation

Sit with your thoughts. Whatever thought arises, send love to that thought.

Mantra meditation

To use the mantra meditation technique you simply silently repeat a mantra over and over. You can use a mala or rosary to help count if you would like. Every time a thought arises, you direct your attention back to the mantra. Research Sanskrit mantras or find an English one that speaks to you. Good mantras: Om; Om Namah Shivaya, Tat tvam asi, Amen; Lord Jesus Christ have mercy on me; Hail Mary, full of grace; I am Loving Awareness, etc.

Chanting meditation

Similar to a mantra meditation, except you say the mantra out loud, and you can sing if you want! Again, whenever thoughts arise, direct your attention back to the mantra.

Breathing meditation

In this technique, your point of focus is your breath. You feel each breath, listen to its sounds, etc. As thoughts arise, you direct your attention back to your breath.

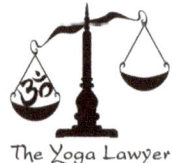
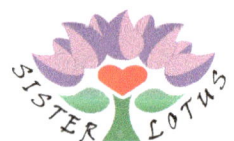

So-hum meditation

Watch your breath. Do not try to control it, just notice it. Feel the breath coming in and out of your nostrils. Notice whether your breath is slow or fast without trying to change it. Listen to the sound of your breath and notice whether it is loud, soft, etc. Using ear plugs facilitates listening to your breath.

Use the "so-hum" mantra to help you focus on your breath: on the "in" breath silently say "so" to yourself. On the "out" breath, silently say, "hum" to yourself. Do this while noticing your breath.

Continue to focus on your breath with the help of the so-hum mantra for 5-10 minutes.

When thoughts pop in your head like, "what am I having for dinner", "what work do I need to do today", or <u>any</u> thought other than your breath, do the following: notice the thought without judging it. Once you notice that you have been involved in a thought, gently bring your awareness back to the "so-hum" mantra and your breath.

Om meditation

For this technique, you listen to the primordial sound, "Om." You might find it most easily accomplished by using ear plugs. Or you can use [Shanmukhi mudra](#). Plug your ears up and listen for any sound. You may hear a sound like what you hear when you listen to a conch shell, or a rustling or buzzing. The sound may sound different today than it does tomorrow. Whatever you hear, go into that sound and listen to it. Feel it resonate in your body. As thoughts arise, turn your attention back to the sound.

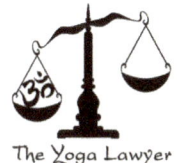

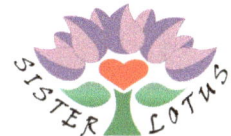

Pratyahara/Bhajan (Eight Limbs cont'd)

Week Seven

Reading:

    SLY Manual "Ashtanga Yoga Chants," pp. 23-8

    SLY Manual "Amma statement on bhajans, the devotional singing," pp. 29-30

Asana, Pranayama, Meditation Practice: Continue to practice asana, pranayama, meditation, or a combination this week. For asana, keep working on the standing postures along with the rest of your Ashtanga "sandwich." Work on the pranayama and meditation practices of your choosing.

Pratyahara Practice: Work to incorporate some pratyahara into your practices this week. That could mean taking extra time and attention in savasana during your asana practice; engaging in sensory deprivation floating; bringing your mind inward from its natural tendency of projection onto external objects back to the internal source of thoughts and emotions (see Byron Katie's "The Work").

Bhajan of Chanting Practice: For your meditation practices this week, be sure to incorporate several sessions of bhajan or chanting out loud. Try to chant for at least 18 repetitions. You can practice the mantras from this manual or a mantra of your choosing. The recording of the Week Six practice of the mantras will be provided to you for reference. Also, several Chants are on YouTube on the YogaLawyer channel, "Yoga Chants" playlist.

Assignment:

1. Research the number 108 and its significance. Why is it a spiritual number and why do people often chant 108 times?

2. Listen to "My Sweet Lord" by George Harrison, and familiarize yourself with the story of the Beatles and Maharishi Mahesh Yogi. Which *two* mantras from the handout are heard near the end of the song?

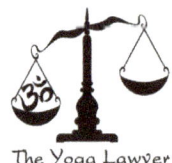

Ashtanga Yoga Chants

Ashtanga Vinyasa Yoga traditionally has both an opening chant and a closing chant. The chants are not overtly religious; they can be performed by those of any religious affiliation.

Because of Yoga's ancient roots, chants, or mantras, are offered in Sanskrit (the ancient language of India). Chanting in another language can help bring the mind into mindfulness, since more concentration is typically required than would be in the chanter's native language. Sanskrit is a language that is said to have been intuited by the ancient Rishis ("seers") based upon the vibratio nal frequency of the words and their objects. It is called "the Mother of all Languages," and English, along with hundreds of other languages, has roots in Sanskrit.

The word mantra comes from two Sanskrit root words: manas, meaning "mind;" and, tra, meaning "protect." Thus, mantras are "mind-protecting."

The chanting or devotional singing ("yoga bhajan") of mantras may shift the consciousness of the individual practitioner to a higher level of vibration. This could be due, in part, to the fact that the mantras have been performed over and over again for thousands of years or more with the same intention, embedding the words themselves with a certain vibratory power.

Mantras are tools for concentration ("dharana") that can lead to states of meditation and mindfulness ("dhyana"). They are practices that can be directly experienced – many practitioners report feelings of peace, love, calmness, and balance. As Amma, "the hugging saint," noted about the practice of the devotional singing of mantras (aka bhajan):

> Bhajans are prayers in the form of songs, rich in meaning and full of devotional content. When one sings a bhajan wholeheartedly, they completely forget themselves and become one with their longing for the divine; this is meditation. In this modern age with distractions galore, traditional meditation and contemplation are not possible for everybody, but anyone can sing bhajans. When sung with concentration and devotion, bhajans awaken the innocence deep within us and we feel the divine in our hearts.

   https://www.amritapuri.org/6773/bhajans.aum <visited June 24, 2021>

Studies have shown that when a person chants it can stabilize their heart rate, lower blood pressure, produce beneficial endorphins in the body and boost metabolic processes. In fact, a recent peer-reviewed study found through MRI tests that chanting "Om" stimulates the vagus nerve, which is associated with heart function, digestion, and physical and mental calmness. Stimulation of the nerve is a treatment for depression, anxiety, epilepsy, migraines, and heart disease, among other conditions, and promotes overall wellbeing. See Int J Yoga. 2011 Jan-Jun; 4(1): 3–6.

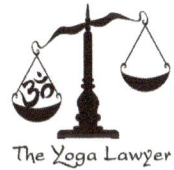

Opening Chant

The Opening chant is a blessing of gratitude offered to the lineage of teachers (including the great Patanjali by name) and their students who have enabled this ancient practice to survive for thousands of years so that we can experience its benefits today. The recitation of this mantra cleanses the energy of the space we have chosen to practice yoga, as well as preparing the mind, body and emotions for the forthcoming Ashtanga Vinyasa sequence.

Om

Vande Gurunam Charanaravinde

Sandarshita Svatma Sukava Bodhe

Nih Sreyase Jangalikyamane

Samsara Halahala Mohashantyai

Abahu Purushakaram

Shankhacakrsi Dharinam

Sahasra Sirasam Svetam

Pranamami Patanjalim

Om

Translation

Om

I bow to the lotus feet of the Supreme Guru

who teaches the great knowledge of the awakening of the happiness of pure Being,

who acts like the jungle physician,

able to eliminate the delusion caused by the poison of conditioned existence (samsara).

I prostrate before the sage Patanjali,

who has thousands of radiant, white heads

and who has, symbolically, assumed the form of a man

holding a conch shell (divine sound), a wheel (discus of light or infinite time) and a sword (discrimination).

Om

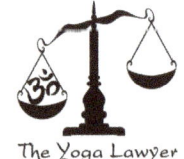
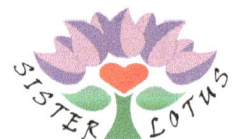

Closing Chant

The Closing Prayer brings the practice to a peaceful end; sealing in the work done and offering the efforts of our practice to improve the state of the world.

Om
Svasthi Praja Bhyaha Pari Pala Yantam
Nya Yena Margena Mahim Mahishaha
Go Brahmanebhyaha Shubamastu Nityam
Lokah Samastah Sukhino Bhavantu
Om Shanti Shanti Shanti
<u>Translation</u>
May prosperity be glorified
May the rulers of the world rule with virtue and justice
May divinity and perfect knowledge be protected
May all beings everywhere be happy and free
Om peace, peace, perfect peace

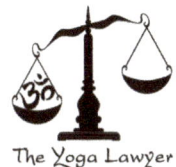
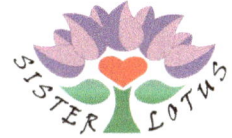

Other important chants/mantras

Shanti mantras

The Shanti mantras come from the Upanishads – a collection of texts at the end of the Vedas (another collection of texts). Also known as Vedanta ("end of the Vedas"), the Upanishads form the basis of the Hindu religion. There are over 200 Upanishads.

Shanti mantra from the Taittiriya, Katha and Shvetashvatara Upanishads

It refers to the student/teacher relationship. It is good to chant at the beginning of a lesson:

Om Sahanaa Vavatu Sahanau Bhunaktu
Saha Veeryam Karavaavahai
Tejasvi Naavadheetamastu Maa Vidvishaavahai
Om Shanti Shanti Shantihi

Translation

May the divine protect us together
May it nourish us together
May we work together and our study be radiant and purposeful
May there be no animosity between us
Om peace, peace, perfect peace

Shanti mantra from the Brihadaranyaka Upanishad:

Om Asato Ma Sadgamaya
Tamaso Ma Jyotirgamaya
Mritor Ma Amritamgamaya
Om Shanti Shanti Shantihi

Translation

Lead us from the unreal to the real
From darkness to light
From death to immortality
May there be peace, peace, perfect peace

Gayatri Mantra

The Gayatri Mantra comes from the Rig Veda, and is one of the most popular mantras; it is recited by people all over the world in the early morning and evening. If you chant it, you can be sure that someone, somewhere in the world is likely chanting it with you. It is a way of showing reverence to the sun, in its metaphorical form as the divine essence in each of us.

Om Bhur Bhuvah Svaha
Tat Saviturvarenyam
Bhargo Devasya Dhimahi

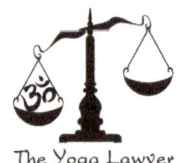
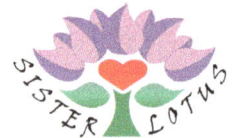

Dhiyo Yo Nah Prachodayat

<u>Translation</u>

Oh Sun (the Divine), may there be peace on the mortal, immortal, and divine plains
I contemplate your brilliant splendor
I pray that it stimulates our intellect and bestows true knowledge

Shiva Shambo

Popular prayer to Shiva, which can be thought of as the divine essence inside of each of us. It can also be thought of as your chosen identifying form of God. For some it is God the Father, or Jesus Christ, or the Divine Mother, or any of a host of other forms.

Shiva Shiva Shiva Shambho
Hare Hare Hare Shambho
(two times)
Mahadeva Shambho Mahadeva Shambho
(two times)

<u>Translation</u>

I worship Shiva, giver of happiness
Praise Shiva
Praise to the Great One, Shiva

Ganesh Prayer

Vakratunda Mahakaya
Kotisurya Samaprabha
Nirvighnam Kurume Deva
Sarvakaryeshu Sarvada

<u>Translation</u>

Lord Ganesh,
with twisted trunk and fat body,
And the brilliance of 100,000 suns,
Please make all my works free of obstacles, always.

Hare Krishna

Hare Krishna (2)
Krishna Krishna, Hare Hare
Hare Rama (2)
Rama Rama, Hare Hare

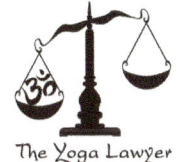
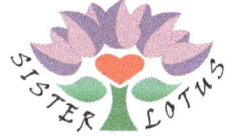

<u>Translation</u>
Praise God
May I reach God

Guru Mantra

Gurur Brahma
Gurur Vishnu
Gururdevo Mahaswarah
Gurur Satkshat Parabrahma
Tasmayi Shree
Guruve Namaha

<u>Translation</u>

Our creation is that guru (Brahma-the force of creation);

The duration of our lives is that guru (Vishnu-the force of preservation);

Our trials, tribulations, and the death of the body is that guru (Shiva, "devo Maheshwara"-the force of destruction or transformation);

The guru is nearby (Guru Sakshat)

The guru is beyond the beyond (param Brahma);

I make my offering (tasmayi) to the beautiful (shree) remover of my darkness (Guruve), to you I bow (namaha).

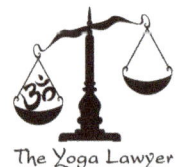
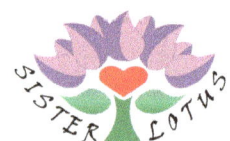

Amma Statement: "Bhajans, the devotional singing"

"Bhajans are prayers in the form of songs, rich in meaning and full of devotional content. When one sings a bhajan wholeheartedly, they completely forget themselves and become one with their longing for the divine; this is meditation. In this modern age with distractions galore, traditional meditation and contemplation are not possible for everybody, but anyone can sing bhajans. When sung with concentration and devotion, bhajans awaken the innocence deep within us and we feel the divine in our hearts."

"While singing the divine name, you should always keep the eyes closed; otherwise, the eyes, persuaded by the mind and tempted by the objects, will run after them. Children, behold the inner light; it cannot be seen if you look at the external light."

"The bliss of singing the divine name is something unique. It is inexpressible. Amma is not at all hesitant to take any number of births to sing the name of the Lord. There is no question of gaining total and complete satisfaction in singing the Lord's name. That is why even those who have reached That State will come down and sing the glories of the Lord with the attitude of a devotee. That is something which one will not feel fed up with at all."

"Darling children, to gain concentration in this age of Kali Yuga (material age), bhajan is easier than meditation. By loud singing, other distracting sounds will be overcome and concentration will be achieved. Bhajan, concentration and meditation, this is the progression. In fact, constant remembrance of God is meditation."

"Children, bhajan sung with one-pointedness will benefit the singer, the listener and also Mother Nature. Such songs will awaken the listeners' minds in due course. If bhajan is sung without concentration, it is a waste of energy. Bhajan is a spiritual discipline aimed at concentrating the mind on one's Beloved Deity. Through that one-pointedness, one can merge in the Divine Being and experience the bliss of one's true self."

"At dusk, the atmosphere is full of impure vibrations. This is the time when day and night meet and is the best time for sadhaks (spiritual aspirants) to meditate because good concentration can be attained. If sadhana is not done, more worldly thoughts rise up. That is why bhajan should be sung loudly at dusk. In this way, the atmosphere will also be purified. Children, at dusk sing bhajan while sitting in front of a burning oil lamp. The smoke produced by the wick burning in oil is a siddha oushadha (perfect medicine). We inhale the smoke and the atmosphere is also purified."

"God alone is eternal. Our life's goal is to attain Him. You should not forget this. Singing the Divine Name is the best way. One should imagine that one's Beloved Deity is standing everywhere in the room. One should pray, 'O Lord, are You not seeing me? O God, please take me on Your lap. I am Your child. I have no one but You as my refuge. Do not abandon me but always dwell in my heart.' Devotional

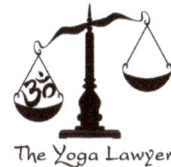

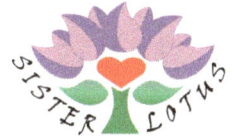

singing is the spontaneous music of the soul. Nobody can resist the inspirational qualities of such music penetrating one's heart when it is sung with concentration and devotion."

"Children, sing from the depth of your hearts. Let the heart melt in prayer. The joy of singing the Lord's name is unique. This bhajan is for us to pour out all our heart's accumulated dirt. Leave aside all shyness and open your hearts to God."

Quote above from Amma, the hugging saint.

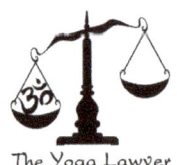
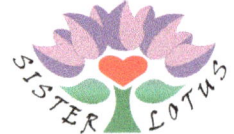

Yoga Sutras

Week Eight

Reading:

Yoga Sutras – Read the preface and introduction from the Mukunda Stiles translation of the Yoga Sutras

Yoga Sutras – read through the first two padas in their entirety – the Samadhi pada and the Sadhana pada. Visit https://www.swamij.com/yoga-sutras.htm for an additional resource.

Also read the parable of the fig tree from the Bible (Mark 11:12-25 and Matthew 21:18-22)

Asana, Pranayama, Meditation Practice: Continue to practice asana, pranayama, meditation (including Bhajan), or a combination this week. Follow the asana videos provided so far, or work on your own Ashtanga "sandwich." Work on the pranayama and meditation practices of your choosing.

Assignment:

1. Check out Masaru Emoto's water experiment and read the parable of the fig tree from the Bible (Mark 11:12-25 and Matthew 21:18-22) and contemplate the power of words.

2. Read the first and second chapter of the Yoga Sutras and identify any sutras you resonate with, would like to understand better, or would just like to look at in more detail. We will be reading through and philosophizing about all the Sutras over the next couple sessions. If you have particular questions that are not covered in the class video, then save them for our discussion during our next one-on-one.

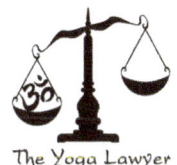
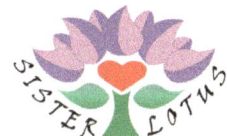

Yoga Sutras Cont'd

Week Nine

Reading:

> Yoga Sutras – Read through the Third Pada, the Vibhuti Pada. Visit https://www.swamij.com/yoga-sutras.htm and see how Swami J groups and organizes all the sutras.

Asana, Pranayama, Meditation Practice: Continue to practice asana, pranayama, meditation (including Bhajan), or a combination this week. For asana, keep working on the standing postures along with the rest of your Ashtanga "sandwich." Follow along with the asana videos provided so far, or do it on your own. Work on the pranayama and meditation practices of your choosing.

Assignment:

1. Read the third chapter of the Yoga Sutras and identify any sutras you resonate with, would like to understand better, or would just like to look at in more detail. We will be reading through and philosophizing about all the Sutras over the next couple sessions. If you have particular questions that are not covered in the class video, then save them for our discussion during our next one-on-one.

2. Look at Swami J's outline for the Third Pada of the Yoga Sutras, the Vibhuti Pada: https://www.swamij.com/yoga-sutras.htm Notice how he groups the sutras and see if that aids understanding.

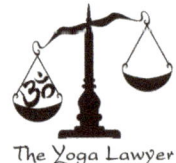

Yoga Sutras Cont'd

Week Ten

<u>Yoga Sutras</u> – Read through the Fourth Pada, the Kaivalya Pada. Visit https://www.swamij.com/yoga-sutras.htm and see how Swami J groups and organizes all the sutras.

<u>Ashtanga Yoga: The Practice Manual</u> by David Swenson, pp. 206-15

<u>Yoga Mala</u> by Sri K. Pattahbi Jois, pp.104-6

<u>Asana, Pranayama, Meditation Practice</u>: Continue to practice asana, pranayama, meditation (including Bhajan), or a combination this week. For asana, we will start adding some more closing postures along to your Ashtanga "sandwich," namely Urdva Dhanarasana (followed by Paschimottanasana A) and Salamba Sarvangasana, and Halasana.

For meditation this week, pick one of the "Samyama" practices from the third pada of the Yoga Sutras and practice it several times throughout the week.

<u>Assignment</u>:

As stated above, for meditation practice this week, you will be picking one of the "Samyama" practices from the third pada of the Yoga Sutras and practicing it several times throughout the week

Review at least 2 or 3 versions of the sutra associated with the Samyama practice that you choose (https://www.swamij.com/yoga-sutras.htm is a great resource).

Translate each word of that sutra, and then come up with a translation of the whole sutra that makes the most sense to you.

You can do it front and back on a note card like the attached examples, or just write it out on a piece of paper or type it up on your computer.

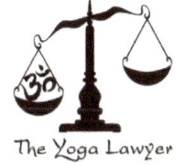

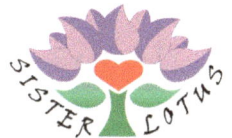

Examples: Front of note cards for sutras III-53, and III-55 containing the Sanskrit version of the sutras and the sutra number.

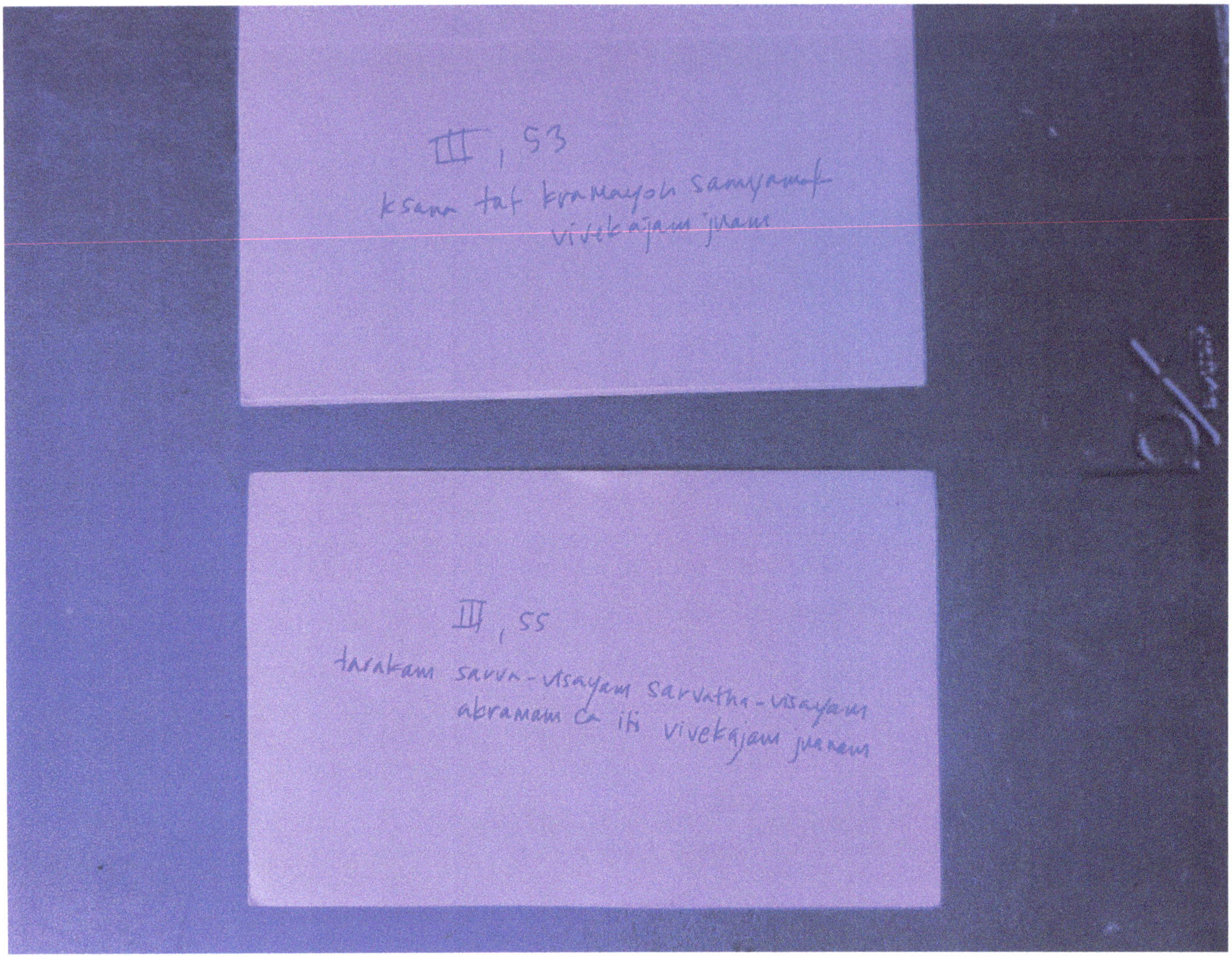

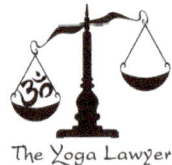
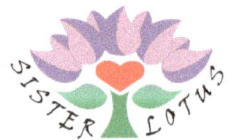

Back of note cards for sutras III-53, III-55 containing the translation of the whole sutra on top in quotes, and the word-for-word translation underneath.

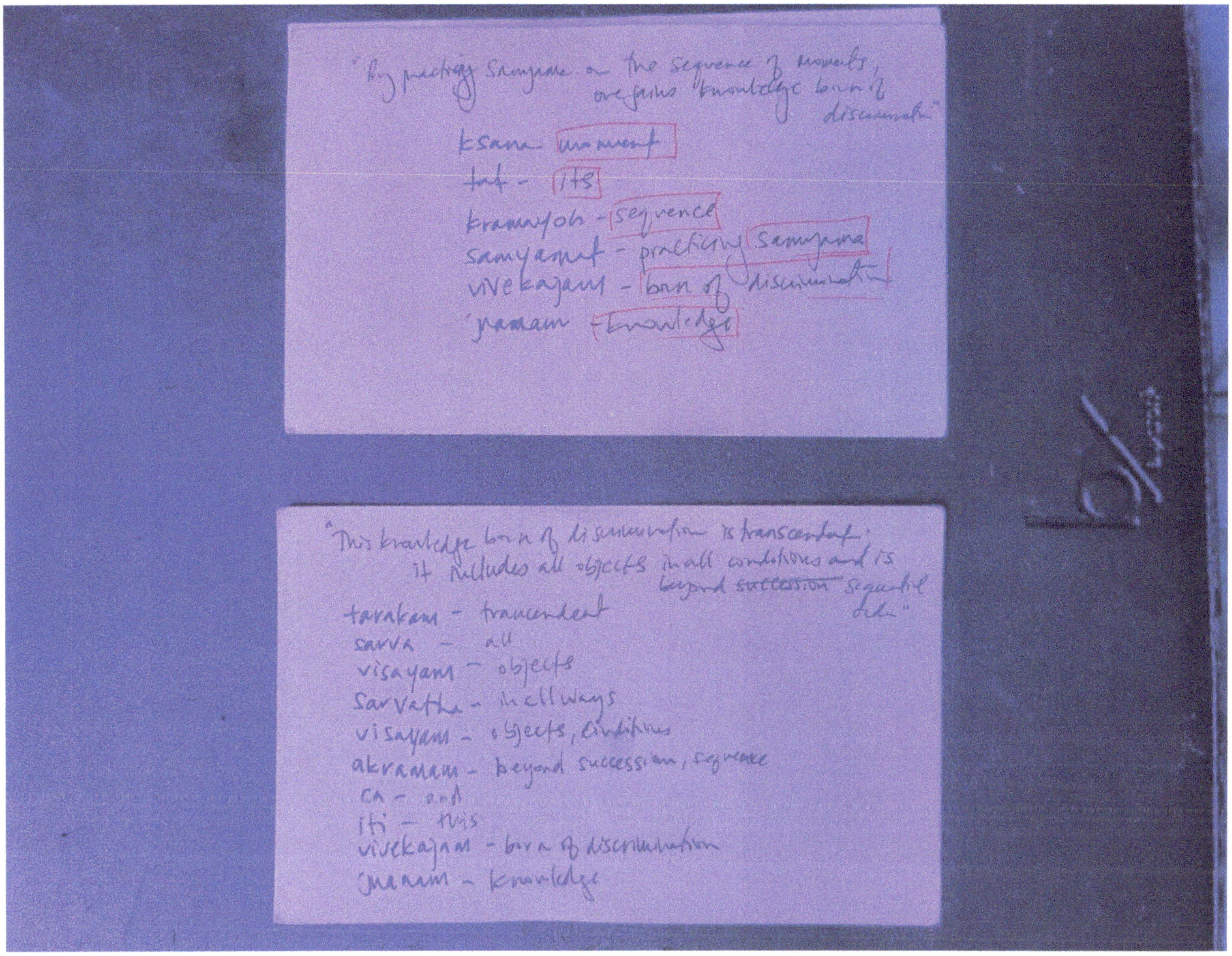

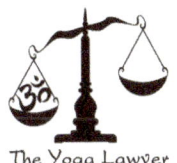
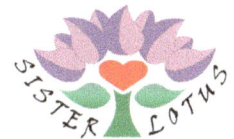

Yoga Anatomy

Week Eleven

Reading/Video

    Watch the Yoganatomy DVDs Volume 1 and 2 with David Keil

Asana, Pranayama, Meditation Practice: Continue to practice asana, pranayama, meditation (including Bhajan), or a combination this week. For asana, keep working your Ashtanga "sandwich." Try to get into a regular groove of practicing asana three (3) times a week (even if only 15 minutes), and doing the other practices more often.

Assignment:

1. Watch the Yoganatomy DVDs Volumes 1 and 2 and take notes of key terms and information that seems important to you. You can handwrite or type your notes. Take a picture or save a copy of your notes and send it to me. You won't be graded on the quality of your notes, this is just for accountability purposes to show that you worked through and immortalized the information in the DVDs in your own way (example attached).

2. Do the partner exercise (with or without a partner) around the 44 minute mark in Volume 1 DVD;

3. Do the asana exercise examples in the Volume 2 DVD within your level of comfort and limitations, skipping or modifying as necessary.

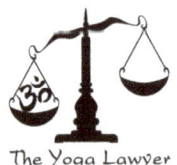
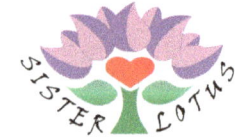

Example: Notes from Volume 1 of Yoganatomy DVD

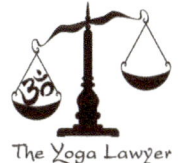
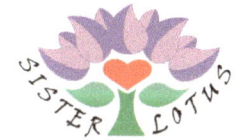

Yoga Anatomy

Week Twelve

Reading/Video

    Watch the Anatomy for Yoga DVD set (11 videos) with Paul Grilley

Asana, Pranayama, Meditation Practice: Continue to practice asana, pranayama, meditation (including Bhajan), or a combination this week. For asana, keep working your Ashtanga "sandwich." Try to get into a regular groove of practicing asana three (3) times a week (even if only 15 minutes), and doing the other practices more often.

Assignment:

    Watch the Anatomy for Yoga DVD set and take notes of key terms and information that seems important to you. You can handwrite or type your notes. Take a picture or save a copy of your notes and send it to me. You won't be graded on the quality of your notes, this is just for accountability purposes to show that you worked through and immortalized the information in the DVDs in your own way (example attached).

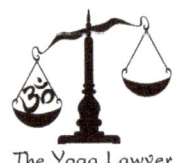
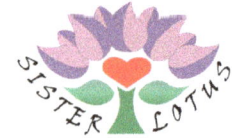

Yoga Anatomy/Adjustments

Week Thirteen

Reading/Video

Watch the Hands on Adjustment videos (2 videos) with David Keil

Asana, Pranayama, Meditation Practice: Continue to practice asana, pranayama, meditation (including Bhajan), or a combination this week. For asana, keep working your Ashtanga "sandwich." Try to get into a regular groove of practicing asana three (3) times a week (even if only 15 minutes), and doing the other practices more often.

Assignment:

1. Watch the Hands on Adjustment DVD set;

2. Pick a few postures that you would like to practice adjustments with and either:
    a. Find a partner at home and try them out (making sure to ask for feedback from your partner);
    b. Come into Total Zen and set up a time to practice adjustments with Kelli; or,
    c. Arrange a remote session with Kelli to go over adjustments.

3. Before next week, obtain a copy of the Bhagavad Gita. One good translation is "the Living Gita" by Sri Swami Satchidananda.

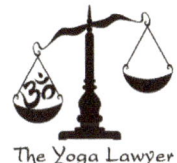
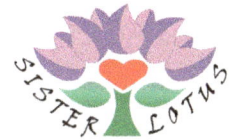

Bhagavad Gita

Week Fourteen

Reading

Read the first six chapters of the Bhagavad Gita. You do not need to have the commentary, just the actual text.

Read the "story behind the Bhagavad Gita" from the Living Gita pp. xi-xvi, also found here: https://integralyogamagazine.org/the-story-behind-the-bhagavad-gita-2/

Asana, Pranayama, Meditation Practice: Continue to practice asana, pranayama, meditation (including Bhajan), or a combination this week. For asana, keep working your Ashtanga "sandwich." Try to get into a regular groove of practicing asana three (3) times a week (even if only 5 minutes of sun salutations), and doing the other practices more often.

Assignment:

1. Read "the story behind the Bhagavad Gita" and the first six (6) chapters of the Bhagavad Gita.

2. Mark or note any slokas (verses) that catch your attention or that you want to look at in more detail.

3. If you still have questions after watching the class video, let's discuss during our next one-on-one! You can also post questions to the Facebook and website community groups.

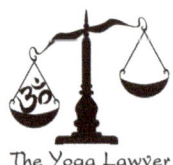
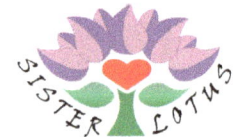

Bhagavad Gita

Week Fifteen

Reading

Read the second six chapters of the Bhagavad Gita (Chapters 7-12). You do not have to read the commentary, just the actual text.

Asana, Pranayama, Meditation Practice: Continue to practice asana, pranayama, meditation (including Bhajan), or a combination this week. For asana, keep working your Ashtanga "sandwich." Try to get into a regular groove of practicing asana three (3) times a week (even if only 5 minutes of sun salutations), and doing the other practices more often.

Assignment:

1. Read the second six (6) chapters (Chapters 7-12) of the Bhagavad Gita.

2. Mark or note any slokas (verses) that catch your attention or that you want to look at in more detail.

3. If you still have questions after watching the class video, let's discuss during our next one-on-one! You can also post questions to the Facebook and website community groups.

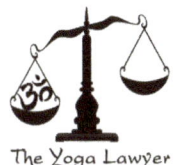
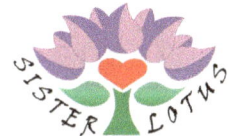

Bhagavad Gita

Week Sixteen

Reading

Read the final six chapters of the Bhagavad Gita (Chapters 13-18). You do not have to read the commentary, just the actual text.

Asana, Pranayama, Meditation Practice: Continue to practice asana, pranayama, meditation (including Bhajan), or a combination this week. For asana, keep working your Ashtanga "sandwich." Try to get into a regular groove of practicing asana three (3) times a week (even if only 5 minutes of sun salutations), and doing the other practices more often.

Assignment:

1. Read the final six (6) chapters (Chapters 13-18) of the Bhagavad Gita to finish it.

2. Mark or note any slokas (verses) that catch your attention or that you want to look at in more detail.

3. If you still have questions after watching the class video, let's discuss during our next one-on-one! You can also post questions to the Facebook and website community groups.

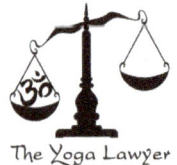

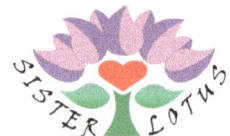

Ayurveda

Week Seventeen

Reading

    SLY Manual "Basic Ayurvedic Principles," pp. 44-6

    "Daily Routine" handout

    "Introduction to Ayurveda" ebook by Banyan Botanicals

    Take a dosha quiz -   https://chopra.com/dosha-quiz

                              https://www.banyanbotanicals.com/info/dosha-quiz/

                              or something similar

Asana, Pranayama, Meditation Practice: Continue to practice asana, pranayama, meditation (including Bhajan), or a combination this week. For asana, keep working your Ashtanga "sandwich." Try to get into a regular groove of practicing asana three (3) times a week (even if only 5 minutes of sun salutations), and doing the other practices more often.

Assignment:

1. Read the handouts and ebook listed above.

2. Take a dosha quiz and determine your Ayurvedic prakriti or constitution.

3. After reading the materials and taking the dosha quiz, note any current, chronic, or seasonal imbalances in your body.

4. Do some research and identify one herb or herb combination that may be beneficial to you based on any imbalance you may have (some common ones that help a lot of common imbalances are Turmeric, Ashwaganda, and Triphala). Start experimenting with that herb in your own body. If you need some guidance in this regard, reach out.

4. Be prepared to discuss your dosha, imbalances, and herb choice at our next one-on-one. You can also post questions to the Facebook and website community groups.

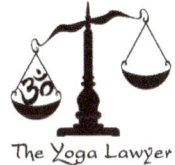

Basic Ayurvedic principles

- The three Doshas[3] also correspond to cycles of the day based upon the natural circadian rhythm of the human body:
  6:00AM – 10:00AM – Kapha
  10:00AM – 2:00 PM – Pitta
  2:00PM – 6:00 PM – Vatta
  6:00 PM – 10:00 PM – Kapha
  10:00PM – 2:00 AM – Pitta
  2:00AM – 6:00 AM – Vatta

- Ideally arise before 6:00 AM (7:00AM DST) to avoid the heaviness and dullness associated with arising during Kapha.

- The longer you sleep past 6:00 AM (7:00AM DST), the worse the possible effect of the Kapha influence throughout the day. You might note that you feel sleepy and dull all day when arising too late in the Kapha period.

- Go to bed by 10:00 PM (11:00 PM DST) to avoid the alertness associated with Pitta.

- The longer you wait to go to bed past 10:00 PM (11:00 PM DST), you might notice the more awake you feel, and the harder it is to fall asleep.

- Your heaviest meal of the day is usually best taken during Pitta when the digestive fires (and digestive enzymes) are strongest and when your hunger is peaking. It should preferably be taken around the early/middle of Pitta.

- It is recommended to do exercise during Kapha periods.

- Your morning meal may be very light or skipped altogether – fruits, fruit juices, green drinks, light cereal (best with non-dairy), toast with nut butter and honey, etc. You will probably find that you do not need much breakfast once you implement these changes.

- Lunch may be heavier. If you want to "cheat" on your healthy diet, for example, and eat cheesecake or pizza or something else "bad," do it in the middle of the day and it will have the least effect on your body weight and digestion.

- Dinner may also be light. Good dinners are simple grains and vegetables, soups and bread, cereal, beans or kitchari, etc.

- Choose whole, organic, GMO-free, and unprocessed foods over their counterparts.

---

[3] For more information on the doshas and for a dosha quiz check out: http://doshaquiz.chopra.com/

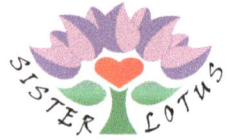

- However, note the effect gluten may have on your digestion. If you are gluten sensitive, you might want to avoid gluten at night. There are amazing substitutes, including rice pastas and millet and other gluten-free breads. To test gluten sensitivity, cut it out of your diet for at 5-7 days. Then "test" yourself by eating something gluten-heavy and noting how your body feels afterward and the next morning upon waking.

- Consider testing for sensitivity/digestibility of these foods: meat, dairy, soy, potatoes, and nightshades (eggplant, tomatoes, and their relatives).

- If you have difficulty digesting certain foods, you might want to limit them and/or maximize their digestibility. Digestibility can be maximized by eating with reverence, eating at midday and when hunger is peaking, and by following the recommended eating order (see next bullet point, below).

- It is recommended to follow the basic Ayurvedic taste principles:
    - The body digests food in the same order it is tasted: sweet, salty, spicy, bitter, astringent
    - Thus, sweet foods should be eaten first, followed by salty, spicy, bitter, and astringent.
    - Milk, cheese, grains, sugar, bread are all sweet foods.
    - Salty foods are anything that tastes salty.
    - Spicy foods are garlic, peppers, ginger, and anything spicy
    - Legumes, and vegetables fall into the bitter and astringent categories.
    - Certain fruits like apples and pomegranates are astringent and are good for dessert
    - The easiest way to figure this out is to eat the heavier foods first, followed by lighter foods. For example, if you are going to eat pizza and salad, eat the pizza first and then the salad. If you eat this during the middle of the day, you will probably notice that it has little to no effect on your weight to eat pizza.
    - Eat dessert first
    - Eat salads last

- Fruit can be eaten any time of day, including dessert (with astringent fruits making the best desserts), but preferably 2 hours after the prior meal (and not to eat again for 2 hours afterward). If 2 hours is too long, you may find even waiting a half an hour aids digestion. It is best to eat fruit by itself, without combining it with other foods.

- Wait 4-6 hours after a meal before eating a new meal. That way, you can be sure that the prior meal was properly digested and that the digestive fires have had a chance to build back up.

- If you get hungry between meals, eat fruit or a hot beverage.

- You will notice that you feel hunger pains in your stomach when it is time for the next meal. This is the "digestive fire" according to Ayurveda. Ayurveda recommends eating only when you feel the digestive fire.

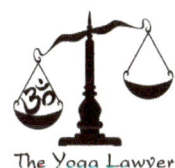

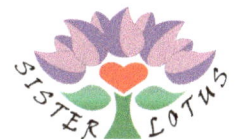

- Sip hot water or tea throughout the day when possible. The amount is not as important as the frequency. According to Ayurveda, this technique helps to dissolve Ama, a sticky substance that is left behind when food is not properly digested, from the body. Ayurveda says that a build up of Ama leads to numerous disorders, including heart disease.

- Chew your food thoroughly and do not talk while chewing. Dr. Vasant Lad recommends chewing each bite 32 times.

- Concentrate on really tasting and enjoying every bite of food. Be mindful while eating. If you are devotional in nature, imagine eating as a form communion with the divine. If you eat meat, think about showing respect and reverence toward the animal you are consuming and recognizing the karmic connection you share.

- Eat slowly.

- Do not eat while under stress or while angry. Instead, spend a few minutes listening to your breath and getting centered before eating.

- Avoid "business lunches" and other stressful events over food.

- Ideally, sit calmly for five minutes before starting to eat. After eating, spend a few minutes just sitting and relaxing before going back to your day.

- Avoid cold beverages. Ask for drinks at restaurants without ice. Cold beverages freeze the digestive track and make digestion more difficult.

- Wait to drink a beverage until after you are done eating. If you have difficulty doing this, at least wait until you are halfway done with your meal before starting to drink a beverage. Drinks dilute the digestive enzymes and make proper digestion of food more difficult.

- Dr. Lad recommends a "thirds" approach to eating: your stomach should be full 1/3 with food, 1/3 with liquid and 1/3 empty after each meal.

- If the above changes seem overwhelming, start with one principle at a time and implement it for a week or more. Once you have that principle under control, add another. You will find it gets easier and easier to do as you go along.

- Above all: Ayurveda teaches that even poison can become nectar if digested properly; and digestion begins in the mind. Eat mindfully and with reverence, above all, and forgive yourself of your poor choices quickly.

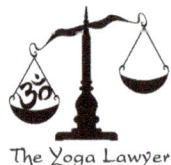
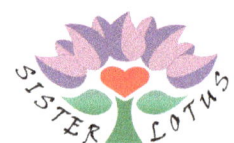

Business of Yoga

Week Eighteen

Reading

    Read the Yoga Alliance's new Ethical Commitment: www.yogaalliance.org/Our_Standards/The_Ethical_Commitment and click on and read the links for the Code of Conduct, Scope of Practice, and Equity in Yoga.

    SLY Manual "Sample Release for Yoga Retreat" – pp. 48-51

Asana, Pranayama, Meditation Practice: Continue to practice asana, pranayama, meditation (including Bhajan), or a combination this week. For asana, keep working your Ashtanga "sandwich." Try to get into a regular groove of practicing asana three (3) times a week (even if only 5 minutes of sun salutations), and doing the other practices more often.

Ayurveda Practice: Incorporate one or more of the practices from the suggested daily routine handouts (like drinking water in the morning or tongue scraping, for example). Continue to experiment with herbs to help balance your doshas.

Assignment:

1. In class, we will be discussing the business of yoga, including these topics:
    a. Yoga Alliance
    b. Yoga Alliance Ethical Commitment
    c. Business ethics
    d. Professionalism (timeliness, consistency, cleanliness)
    e. Insurance
    f. Waivers/Releases
    g. Incorporating in Florida
    h. Federal tax id number
    i. Invoicing
    j. Marketing and Promotion
    k. Continuing education

2. Try to familiarize yourself with the above topics, including reading the Yoga Alliance guidelines as set forth above, prior to watching the class video.

5. Review the topics ahead of class and think of any questions you might have or other business topics you want to discuss during a one-on-one or to the Facebook and website community groups.

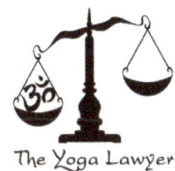

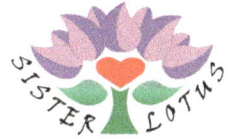

SAMPLE RELEASE FOR YOGA RETREAT

Liability Release, Waiver, and Assumption of Risk

I, _____, enter this Liability Release, Waiver and Assumption of Risk ("Waiver") with Nameless Yoga Retreats. As I enter this Waiver, I acknowledge that all parties involved are setting our intentions that only good will come of this contractual union, and that all parties and the Universe will benefit. I agree as follows:

I. **FOREIGN TRAVEL WAIVER**

I acknowledge that travel to foreign countries may involve many risks not known to me or to Nameless Yoga Retreats, ABC, LLC, Sister Lotus Yoga, YogaLawyer, and their owners, operators, officers, employees, independent contractors, representatives, agents, or anyone else attending or participating in a Retreat or other Program. These risks may not be reasonably foreseeable at this time or at the time of the Retreat or Program in which I participate, and may not normally be associated with travel. I knowingly and voluntarily agree to assume any and all risks associated with such travel.

II. **ASSUMPTION OF RISK**

I am aware of and hereby acknowledge the inherent risks associated with Retreat or Program activities, including, but not limited to, the risks associated with yoga, dance, art, hoop, poi, transformative experiences, mountain nature excursions, hiking, swimming, foreign travel, and any other activities associated with the Retreat or Program I am attending. I am aware of the risks of injury, death, and property damage that may result from, among other causes, the acts or omissions of Nameless Yoga Retreats, ABC, LLC, Sister Lotus Yoga, YogaLawyer, and their owners, operators, officers, employees, independent contractors, representatives, and/or agents. I further assume all risks associated with my participation in the Retreat or Program including, without limitation, the risk of negligent or intentional acts or omissions or theft by other participants or third parties, and the risk of injury caused by the condition of any property, facilities or equipment used during the Retreat or Program.

III. **RELEASE OF LIABILITY**

I, in exchange for $100 (included in the total payment for the Retreat or Program), voluntarily and while realizing the full legal significance of my action, waive and release, on behalf of myself, my heirs and my estate, all claims of whatever nature against Nameless Yoga Retreats, ABC, LLC, Sister Lotus Yoga, YogaLawyer, and their owners, operators,

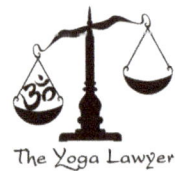

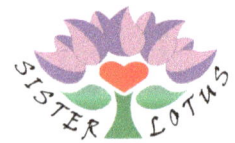

officers, employees, independent contractors, representatives, and/or agents including, but not limited to, claims of any injury, loss, damage, accident, delay, irregularity or expense caused by strikes, war, weather, sickness, quarantine, government restrictions, or arising from any act or omission of any steamship, airline, railroad, bus company, hotel, restaurant, school or university, firm, agency or individual, or for any other cause whatsoever arising out of, resulting from or in connection with the Retreat or Program.

IV. <u>INDENMINFICATION AND HOLD HARMLESS</u>

It is expressly understood and agreed that Nameless Yoga Retreats is not providing personal chaperones or supervision with respect to this Retreat or Program and that I am responsible for my individual conduct, health and safety at all times. I agree to defend, indemnify and hold harmless Nameless Yoga Retreats, ABC, LLC, Sister Lotus Yoga, YogaLawyer, and their owners, operators, officers, employees, independent contractors, representatives, and/or agents for any and all demands, costs, losses, expenses, claims, recoveries, judgments and liabilities (including attorneys' fees) of any nature arising out of, or in consequence of, my acts, words, conduct, etc. in any way connected with my participation in the Retreat or Program including, but not limited to, damage to property, any injuries or death sustained by any person(s).

V. <u>MODIFICATION OF PROGRAM</u>

I understand that the remoteness of the destination, local custom, political upheaval or other political issues and/or prevailing weather conditions may cause minor inconvenience or modification to portions of the Retreat or Program. Nameless Yoga Retreats reserves the right to modify and/or cancel any tour arrangements due to reasonable circumstances.

VI. <u>TRAVEL DOCUMENTS</u> AND INSURANCE

I understand that it is my responsibility to ensure that all necessary travel documents such as passports (at least six (6) months prior to expiration date), visas, and yoga qualifications (if applicable) are obtained and are valid.

I understand that Nameless Yoga Retreats reserves the right to require travel insurance for any Retreat or Program and further recommends travel insurance for all Retreats or Programs. Obtaining travel insurance is my responsibility and Nameless Yoga Retreats is not liable for any damages arising from my failure to obtain travel insurance.

VII. <u>REPRESENTATION OF GOOD HEALTH</u>

I am in good health, have no physical conditions that affect my ability to travel and/or participate in any of the activities involved in this Retreat or Program, and I have not been advised otherwise by a medical practitioner. I acknowledge that Nameless Yoga Retreats is in no way responsible for any costs related to my medical care.

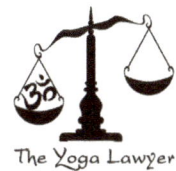
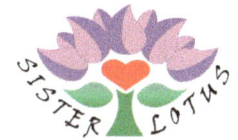

VIII. CHOICE OF LAW; VENUE

This Waiver shall be governed by the laws of the State of Colorado, USA. The parties agree that any lawsuit brought to enforce the terms of this Waiver and/or to recover any alleged damages arising from this Waiver or from participation in a Retreat or Program must be filed in the Trial Court of Colorado in and for _____ County, and each of the parties consents to the jurisdiction of such court (and of the appropriate appellate courts) in any such action or proceeding and waives any objection to such venue.

IX. BROAD CONSTRUCTION;

This Waiver is a legally binding agreement and will be construed broadly to provide a release and waiver to the maximum extent permissible under applicable law.

X. ENFORCEABILITY

If any provision of this Waiver is held by a court of competent jurisdiction to be invalid or unenforceable, the reminder of the Waiver shall remain in full force and effect and shall in no way be impaired.

XI. KNOWING AND VOLUNTARY EXECUTION

I acknowledge that I have carefully read this Waiver, understand its contents, and understand that this Waiver includes a release of liability and an assumption of the risk. I acknowledge that Nameless Yoga Retreats is materially relying on this waiver and is allowing you to engage in activities including but not limited to yoga, dance, art, hoop, poi, transformative experiences, and mountain nature excursions, etc.

XII. USE OF PICTURES AND VIDEOS

Nameless Yoga Retreats may use any pictures or videos taken of participants during the Retreat or Program. This includes digital images which may be posted on our website. By participating in any Nameless Yoga Retreats Retreat or Program, I agree that I am consenting to the use of my image or likeness by Nameless Yoga Retreats for any purpose, including but not limited to electronic and printed promotional material.

XIII. DISCLOSURE OF PERTINENT INFORMATION

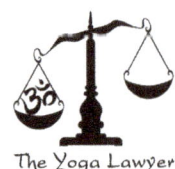
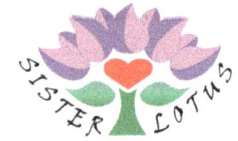

It is essential that any pertinent information, including any social, emotional or physical problems that might limit your active participation in Nameless Yoga Retreats' Retreats or Programs be discussed with the directors prior to acceptance and attendance in a Retreat or Program. We want this to be a successful experience for the participant and Nameless Yoga Retreats.

Caution: this is a release of legal rights. Read and understand it before signing.

Signature _____ Date _____

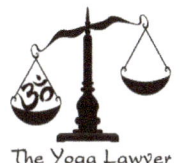
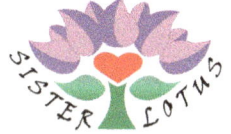

Teaching Methodology

Week Nineteen

<u>Reading</u>

No reading this week

<u>Asana, Pranayama, Meditation Practice</u>: Continue to practice asana, pranayama, meditation (including Bhajan), or a combination this week. For asana, keep working your Ashtanga "sandwich." Try to get into a regular groove of practicing asana three (3) times a week (even if only 5 minutes of sun salutations), and doing the other practices more often.

<u>Ayurveda Practice</u>: Incorporate one or more of the practices from the suggested daily routine handouts (like drinking water in the morning or tongue scraping, for example). Continue to experiment with herbs to help balance your doshas.

<u>Assignment</u>:

1. In class, we will be discussing teaching methodology, including these topics:
    a. Ashtanga Vinyasa methodology
        i. Tristhana
        ii. Vinyasa
        iii. Lineage recognition –
            1. Beginning
            2. End
            3. Namaste?
    b. Sequencing
        i. Traditional primary series
        ii. Ashtanga Sandwich
        iii. Other limbs
    c. Pacing
        i. Self-paced
        ii. Count
        iii. Breath
    d. Environment
        i. Safe
        ii. Accessible
        iii. Welcoming
    e. Cueing
        i. Verbal
        ii. Visual
        iii. Physical
    f. Class management

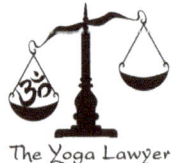

          i. Different skill levels
          ii. Mysore-style v. Led
    g. Different types of classes:
          i. Asana
          ii. Pranayama
          iii. Philosophy
          iv. Other limbs
          v. What else?
    h. Workshops

6. Review the topics ahead of class and watch the video. If you have questions after watching the class video, let's discuss during our next one-on-one! You can also post questions to the Facebook and website community groups.

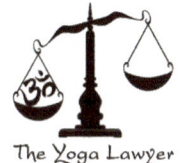

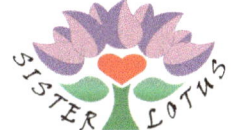

Practicum/Graduation

Week Twenty

As discussed in the class video, the Practicum can be completed anytime and is required before you will get your certificate of completion. The practicum requires you to fill out the self-assessment, below, and to get two (2) students to perform the evaluations, below.

In addition to the Practicum, there were a handful of "accountability" assignments during the course. Use the "Required Assignments" checklist on page 69, below, to make sure you have all the requirements to complete the course.

Once you have completed the checklist, you will receive your certificate.

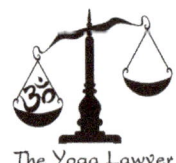
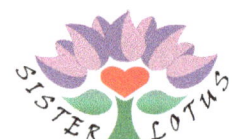

Practicum

Class Description: Describe the class you are teaching. Is it pranayama, asana, meditation, a combination, or something else? What would you call your class if it was taught at a Yoga studio?

Specific practices: Outline your class framework and list the specific practices you will be teaching. If you are teaching an asana-focused class, state which asanas you are teaching (including the Sanskrit names!); if its pranayama, describe the pranayama techniques; if its chanting, describe the chants; if it's a hybrid, describe that, etc.

Self-critique: How did you do? What went well? What could you do better next time?

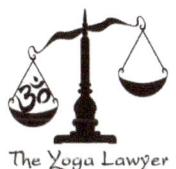
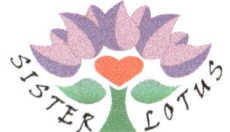

Student Evaluation

Name:

Date:

How would you rate your yoga class on a scale of 1-10?

What positive or constructive feedback can you offer?

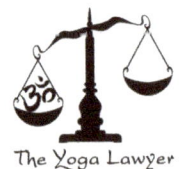

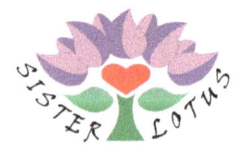

Student Evaluation

Name:

Date:

How would you rate your yoga class on a scale of 1-10?

What positive or constructive feedback can you offer?

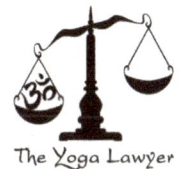

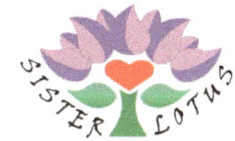

Outside Yoga Class Worksheet

As part of your 200-hour RYT Apprenticeship Program, you will be attending a yoga class offered by a teacher unaffiliated with Sister Lotus Yoga. You can attend in person or online, and it can be just about any type of yoga class – including Kundalini, Hatha, Bikram, etc. Use this form to evaluate the class that you choose. Please complete before the end of your training program.

Name of class:

Teacher:

Date:

Length of class:

What was the format of the class?: (i.e., was it like our Ashtanga yoga "sandwich" with warm-up, standing, seated, backbending, inversions, closing? Or was it different?)

What did you like about the class? Was there anything you disliked?

What could you apply from the class in your own teaching practice?

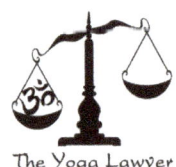

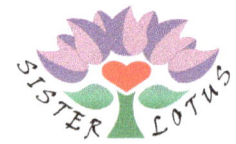

Required Assignments check list

- ☐ Miracle of Mindfulness short summary (week 6)

- ☐ Yoga Sutra note card (week 10)

- ☐ Yoga Anatomy notes (week 11)

- ☐ Yoga Anatomy notes (week 12)

- ☐ Practicum worksheet (week 19)

- ☐ Student evaluation 1 (week 19)*

- ☐ Student evaluation 2 (week 19)*

- ☐ Outside yoga class worksheet (week 19)

*if you have difficulty getting your two (2) students to do an evaluation, you can alternatively take a picture or screenshot of them taking your class.

"O Arjuna! The yogi is thought to be greater than the ascetic, greater than the learned, and greater than the man of action; therefore be a yogi!" ~ Chapter 6:46, Bhagavad Gita

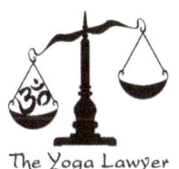
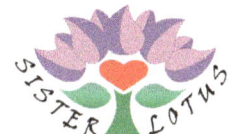

Notes

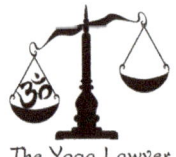

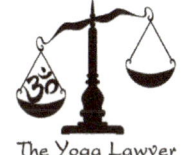
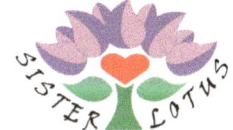

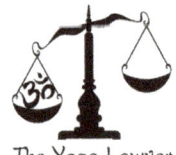
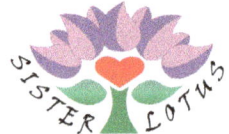

www.ingramcontent.com/pod-product-compliance
Lightning Source LLC
Chambersburg PA
CBHW040223040426
42333CB00051B/3426